Type 2 Diabetes
BASICS

D1462429

Patti Rickheim, MS, RN, CDE
Jill Flader, MS, RD, CDE
with
Karol M. Carstensen

INTERNATIONAL DIABETES CENTER

Minneapolis

Type 2 Diabetes BASICS is an education program for people who are not treated with insulin. This book is designed to be used as part of the program, which is usually taught by a certified diabetes educator (CDE). It is divided into four sections to coincide with the four sessions of the program. The sessions are sequenced as follows:

Session 1: As scheduled
Session 2: Two weeks after Session 1
Session 3: Three months after Session 1
Session 4: Three months after Session 3

Readers may choose to use this book as a reference outside of the program format. However, it is strongly advised that all people with diabetes seek appropriate medical care and diabetes education from trained healthcare professionals.

International Diabetes Center
3800 Park Nicollet Boulevard
Minneapolis, MN 55416-2699
888-825-6315
www.idcpublishing.com

Copy Editor: Rosemary Wallner
Production Manager: Gail Devery
Cover and Text Design: Fruitful Results
Text Production: David Enyeart
Illustrations: John Bush

ISBN 1-885115-54-7

Printed in the United States of America

Acknowledgments

The authors would like to thank the Type 2 Diabetes BASICS Team at the International Diabetes Center, Minneapolis, for their commitment to the program and to our clients.

Peggy Baldy

Susan Beck, BSN, RN

Richard M. Bergenstal, MD, Executive Director

Nancy Cooper, RD, LD, CDE

Janet Davidson, BSN, RN, CDE

Tamara Eiden

Deb Elsen, BSN, RN, CDE

Colleen Fischer, RD, LD, CDE

Cathy Johnson, RN

David Kendall, MD, Medical Director

Allison Martinson

Betsy Moga, BSN, RN

Jan Pearson, BAN, RN, CDE

Gail Radosevich, RD, LD

Diane Reader, RD, LD, CDE

Kathy Reynolds, RN, CDE

Jennifer Robinett, BSN, RN

Angela Sharp, MPH, RD, LD, CDE

Joy Smetanka, RD, CDE

Brenda Solarz-Johnson, BSN, RN, CDE

Sue Sorenson, RD, LD

TABLE OF CONTENTS

Welcome

In this session, you will:

- gain an understanding of diabetes and what causes it

- learn how diabetes is treated and the goals of treatment

- discover the importance of controlling blood glucose levels

- learn how food planning and physical activity enhance diabetes control

- learn about carbohydrate foods and how they affect your blood glucose levels

- learn the importance of regular physical activity

- learn how and when to test your blood glucose

- begin to feel better about your ability to manage diabetes

What Is Diabetes?

Diabetes is a condition that causes high blood glucose (blood sugar) levels. It is a chronic disease that can be managed but not cured. It doesn't go away.

Proper diabetes treatment and education can help you stay healthy. You can learn to live well with diabetes. That is our goal.

Without proper treatment, diabetes can cause damage to the large and small blood vessels. Blood vessel damage can lead to serious nerve, heart, eye, or kidney problems. But this doesn't have to happen.

You are taking the first step toward living well with diabetes. Many people will help you along the way. These include your doctor, nurse educators, registered dietitians, other health professionals, and your family and friends. They are all on your team.

Diagnosing Diabetes

Diabetes is diagnosed through blood tests that measure the glucose level in the blood.

- A fasting blood glucose test is done when a person has consumed nothing but water for at least eight hours.

- A casual, or random, blood glucose test can be done at any time.

Two blood tests done on different days are required to diagnose diabetes.

Sometimes blood glucose levels are higher than normal but not high enough to be diabetes. Two conditions cause this. They are impaired fasting glucose and impaired glucose tolerance. People with these conditions are at risk for diabetes. Following the recommendations in this book can help reduce the risk.

DIAGNOSIS	FASTING TEST	CASUAL TEST
Diabetes	126 mg/dL or higher	200 mg/dL or higher (with symptoms)
Impaired fasting glucose or Impaired glucose tolerance	110–125 mg/dL *borderline*	140–199 mg/dL
Normal	110 mg/dL or lower	140 mg/dL or lower

Glucose and Insulin

The food we eat is digested and converted into glucose. Glucose is the body's main energy source. It is carried in the bloodstream to the body's cells. Inside the cells, it is converted into energy.

Insulin helps glucose get into the cells. Insulin is a hormone made in the pancreas. It attaches to cells in the body. Insulin opens the cells to allow glucose to get inside.

Diabetes is caused by a breakdown in this process. Insulin is absent or poorly used. Glucose stays in the bloodstream, and blood glucose levels rise.

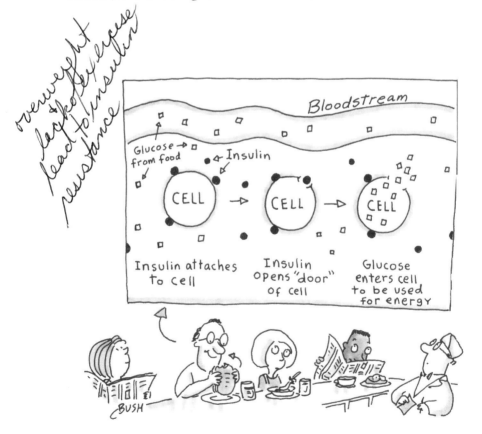

overweight & lack of exercise lead to insulin resistance

Bloodstream

Glucose from food

Insulin

CELL → CELL → CELL

Insulin attaches to cell

Insulin opens "door" of cell

Glucose enters cell to be used for energy

BUSH

6

Types of Diabetes

There are three types of diabetes. Each type occurs for a different reason. All three types of diabetes cause high blood glucose levels.

TYPE 1 DIABETES

The immune system destroys the insulin-producing cells in the pancreas. The cells stop making insulin. This means that the body can't use glucose for energy. People with type 1 diabetes need insulin injections every day to stay alive. Type 1 diabetes can begin at any age. It usually occurs in children or in young adults under age 30.

TYPE 2 DIABETES

The pancreas does not make enough insulin or the body cannot use insulin properly. The body "resists" the action of insulin. Glucose doesn't get into the body's cells very well. Type 2 diabetes is more common in people over age 45, but even children can develop it.

GESTATIONAL DIABETES

The hormonal changes of pregnancy demand more insulin than the body can make. After the birth of the baby, blood glucose levels return to normal in most women. Women who have had gestational diabetes are at risk for developing type 2 diabetes later in life.

Type 2 Diabetes Risk Factors

Many things contribute to a diagnosis of diabetes. Can you answer "yes" to any of the questions on page 9? Your "yes" answers show your risk factors.

Many risk factors are out of your control. For example, you can't change your age or your family history. Understanding your risk factors can help you understand your diagnosis.

Ask your family members to answer the questions, too. They are at risk for diabetes. Steps can be taken now that can help reduce their risk. Two important steps are eating healthfully and staying physically active.

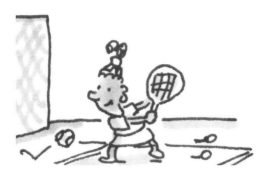

RISK FACTOR ROUND-UP

Answer the questions below. "Yes" answers show your risk factors for diabetes.

Yes	No	
☐	☒	Does someone in your family have diabetes?
☒	☐	Are you over the age of 45?
☒	☐	Are you overweight?
☐	☒	Are you inactive (no regular exercise program)?
☒	☐	Do you have high blood pressure?
☐	☐	Do you have abnormal blood cholesterol or triglycerides?
☐	☒	Do you have a history of diabetes during pregnancy?
☐	☒	Have you had impaired fasting glucose in the past?
☒	☐	Do you now have impaired fasting glucose or impaired glucose tolerance?
☐	☒	Are you African American, American Indian, Hispanic, Asian, Alaska Native, Native Hawaiian, or Pacific Islander?

Symptoms of Diabetes

Diabetes has both "classic" and "common" symptoms. Classic symptoms are usually linked with type 1 diabetes. Common symptoms occur more often with type 2 diabetes. You may have many symptoms or none at all.

Even if you don't have symptoms, it's important to do everything you can to manage your diabetes. Start today!

CLASSIC SYMPTOMS	COMMON SYMPTOMS
Frequent urination	Fatigue
Increased thirst	Blurred vision
Increased hunger	Frequent infections
Unexplained weight loss	Poor wound healing
	Dry, itchy skin
	Numbness and tingling in hands, legs, and feet

Complications of Diabetes

High blood glucose levels can lead to serious health complications. You need to take charge and take care of your diabetes, so this doesn't happen to you.

Blood glucose control helps prevent, delay, or slow the progression of complications. The complications of diabetes include:

- eye problems

- heart and blood vessel disease

- kidney disease

- foot problems

- nerve damage

- sexual dysfunction in men

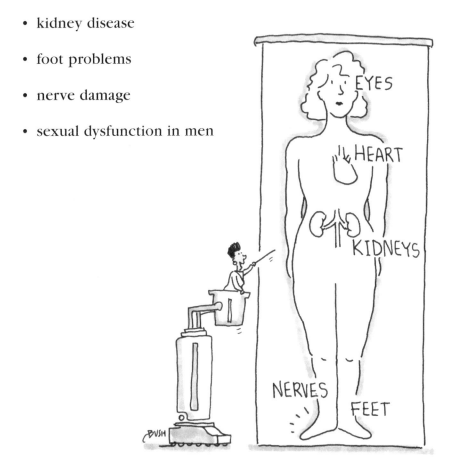

Type 2 Diabetes Treatment

The goals of diabetes treatment are to help you:

- keep blood glucose levels within a target range

- feel better every day

- prevent, delay, or slow the progression of diabetes complications

- balance diabetes management with your lifestyle

Your treatment is based on what your body needs. Diabetes treatment options are shown on the next page. Some people need to take a medication right away. Others start treatment with a food plan and activity alone.

Over time, medications may be added or changed in your treatment plan. Diabetes medications include diabetes pills and insulin injections. Both can help lower blood glucose levels.

The table on pages 90–91 shows the diabetes pills now being used to treat type 2 diabetes. Different diabetes pills work in different ways. They:

- help the pancreas release more insulin

- help the body use insulin better

- make the liver release less glucose

- slow down the absorption of carbohydrates

You need the best treatment for you. The best treatment is the one that keeps your blood glucose levels in control.

DIABETES TREATMENT OPTIONS

Food & Activity Plan

Food & Activity Plan   **+**   Diabetes Pill

Food & Activity Plan   **+**   Diabetes Pill   **+**   Diabetes Pill

Food & Activity Plan   **+**   Diabetes Pill(s)   **+**   Insulin

Food & Activity Plan   **+**   Insulin

13

Blood Glucose Tests

You and your healthcare provider will use two tests to monitor your blood glucose levels. One test is done in a laboratory. The other test you do yourself.

HEMOGLOBIN A$_{1c}$ TEST

During your regular visits, your healthcare provider often will draw a blood sample. The sample is used for a hemoglobin A$_{1c}$ test (HbA$_{1c}$). This test measures your average blood glucose level over the past two months. The value is reported as a percentage (%).

You need to have an HbA$_{1c}$ test every three to four months. The target for HbA$_{1c}$ is no more than 1 to 1.5 percentage points over normal. Ask your healthcare provider to help you fill in the blanks below.

....

The normal range for my provider's lab is _____ to _____ .

My target HbA$_{1c}$ is _____%.

Based on a normal of 6%,   your average blood
if your HbA$_{1c}$ is: glucose level is:

HbA$_{1c}$	Average blood glucose
4%	50
5%	80
6%	115
7%	150
8%	180
9%	210
10%	245
11%	280
12%	310
13%	345

14

SELF BLOOD GLUCOSE TEST

You will learn how to do a simple blood glucose test yourself using a blood glucose meter. You need to test your blood glucose regularly.

A self blood glucose test gives you a "snapshot" of your blood glucose level at the moment you test. Keep a record of the results in your Diabetes Record Book. Your record book holds all your test results—all your snapshots—in one place, like a photo album.

When you look at all the snapshots together, you can see a bigger picture. You see your blood glucose control over time.

Regular testing and record keeping help you and your healthcare provider:

- evaluate your blood glucose control

- decide what changes you may need to make to improve your blood glucose control

- see how the changes affect your blood glucose levels

- determine how well your treatment plan is working

SAMPLE DIABETES RECORD BOOK

Date	3 AM BG	BREAKFAST			LUNCH			DINNER			BEDTIME	
		BG	Med	BG	BG	Med	BG	BG	Med	BG	BG	Med
6-5		179	Glyburide 5mg					138		181		
6-6		156	"					94		138		
6-7		146	"					169		199		

15

Target Blood Glucose Ranges

The target range for self blood glucose tests is a little higher than the normal range. The goal is to have at least one half (50%) of your test results within the target range.

TEST TIME	TARGET RANGE	NORMAL RANGE
Before meals	80–140 mg/dL	70–110 mg/dL
1½ hours after meals	Below 180 mg/dL	Below 140 mg/dL
Bedtime	100–140 mg/dL	Below 120 mg/dL

Sometimes your blood glucose level will be outside the target range. That's okay. Your blood glucose levels don't have to be perfect.

When 50% or more of your tests are within range, your HbA_{1c} will usually be in target too. It may be several weeks after you start your treatment before your HbA_{1c} changes.

Self Blood Glucose Testing Times

When you start out, it is recommended that you do three blood glucose tests every day. The times for testing are:

• before breakfast

• before your main meal

• 1½ hours after your main meal

If you feel you can, commit to testing on this schedule for two weeks. Write your test results in your record book.

Simple Steps for Self Testing

Follow this simple procedure to test your blood glucose level. You will need certain supplies for testing. Your health-care provider can tell you what they are. (See page 92.)

1. Wash hands with soap and water. Dry thoroughly.

2. Put a test strip into the meter.

3. Poke your finger with the lancet.

4. Gently massage the area until a drop of blood forms.

5. Place the blood drop on the test strip.

6. Wait for the test result to be displayed.

7. Record the result in your Diabetes Record Book.

TESTING TIPS

- Change the site each time you poke your finger.

- Use the side of your finger rather than the tip.

- Keep test strips covered, dry, and in packaging until used.

- Follow instructions supplied by the meter manufacturer.

- Dispose of lancets properly. (See page 93.)

- Don't let test strips freeze or overheat.

Your Diabetes Food Plan

Your blood glucose levels are affected by what, when, and how much you eat. Your diabetes treatment includes a food plan. The plan serves as a guide to help you make decisions about food and the timing of meals.

Your diabetes food plan reflects your health needs and how you like to eat. It usually includes three meals and may include snacks. You don't have to eat special foods. There is no strict diabetes diet. You can enjoy all the foods you like and still take care of your diabetes. Your food plan helps you:

- keep blood glucose levels in the target range

- maintain healthy levels of blood cholesterol and triglycerides

- prevent diabetes complications

- maintain a healthy body weight

- eat healthfully

Carbohydrate Foods

Your food plan is focused on carbohydrate foods. Carbohydrate foods include starchy foods, fruit, milk, some milk products, and sweets.

Carbohydrate foods are digested and converted into glucose. Carbohydrate foods make blood glucose levels go up.

But carbohydrate foods are good for you, too! They contain many other important nutrients, vitamins, and minerals. Carbohydrate gives your body energy and supports proper body function.

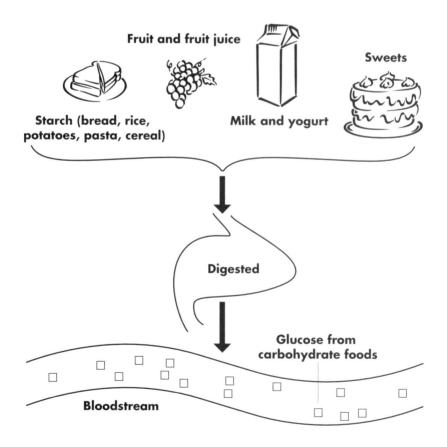

Fruit and fruit juice

Sweets

Starch (bread, rice, potatoes, pasta, cereal)

Milk and yogurt

Digested

Glucose from carbohydrate foods

Bloodstream

Carbohydrate Counting

If you eat too much carbohydrate at one time, you can over-load your insulin supply. Glucose from the carbohydrate backs up in the bloodstream. Your blood glucose level goes up too high.

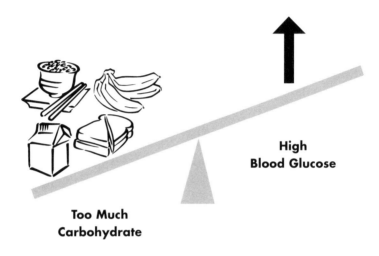

**High
Blood Glucose**

**Too Much
Carbohydrate**

Carbohydrate counting helps you keep track of how much carbohydrate you eat for meals and snacks. It's best to eat small amounts of carbohydrate at different times during the day, rather than a lot at one time. This helps control your blood glucose levels.

WHAT IS A CARBOHYDRATE CHOICE?

One carbohydrate choice is a serving of food that contains about 15 grams of carbohydrate. Your food plan tells you how many choices you have for each meal. You decide which carbohydrate foods you want to eat.

You need to know the correct serving size of foods to count carbohydrates. If you eat double the serving size, you need to count the carbohydrate choices twice.

 = 1 choice (15 grams carbohydrate)

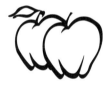 = 2 choices (30 grams carbohydrate)

Count the Carbohydrate

Figure out how many carbohydrate choices are in each sample meal. You can write in a meal of your own on the next page, if you prefer. Refer to My Food Plan or another list of carbohydrate foods with serving sizes to help you count. Can you figure out the fast food meal from the information you have?

BREAKFAST	AMOUNT	CARBOHYDRATE CHOICES
Orange juice	½ cup	1
Cereal, dry	¾ cup	1
Milk	½ cup	½
Eggs	2	
Toast, whole wheat	2 slices	2
Jelly or honey, regular	1 Tbsp	
TOTAL CARBOHYDRATE	=	4½

DINNER	AMOUNT	CARBOHYDRATE CHOICES
Fish, broiled	3 oz	
Rice, cooked	⅔ cup	2
Broccoli, steamed	½ cup	
Bread roll	1 oz or one	1
Margarine	1 tsp	
Ice cream	½ cup	1
Coffee	1 cup	
TOTAL CARBOHYDRATE	=	4

SNACK	AMOUNT	CARBOHYDRATE CHOICES
Popcorn	3 cups	1
TOTAL CARBOHYDRATE	**=**	1

FAST FOOD MEAL	CARBOHYDRATE CHOICES
Big Mac	4
French fries, large	4
16 oz Diet Coke	
MacDonaldland cookies (1 box)	
TOTAL CARBOHYDRATE **=**	

MY TYPICAL MEAL	AMOUNT	CARBOHYDRATE CHOICES
TOTAL CARBOHYDRATE	**=**	

Understanding Food Labels

The nutrition labels on food packages are valuable tools. They give all the information you need for carbohydrate counting.

Look at the label on the next page, then take the food label quiz. Use the chart below as a guide for converting carbohydrate grams to carbohydrate choices.

CARBOHYDRATE GRAMS		CARBOHYDRATE CHOICES
15 grams	=	1 choice
30 grams	=	2 choices
45 grams	=	3 choices
60 grams	=	4 choices
75 grams	=	5 choices

FOOD LABEL QUIZ

What is the serving size of this food? _____ 1 cup

How many servings are in this package? _____ 2

How many grams of carbohydrate does this food contain? 31

One serving of this food counts as _____ 2 _____ carbohydrate choices.

Answers: 1 cup; 2; 31; 2

24

SERVING SIZE

All the information on the label is based on this portion. If you eat double the serving size, you will eat double the carbohydrate, other nutrients, and calories.

Nutrition Facts

Serving Size 1 cup (228g)
Servings Per Container 2

Amount Per Serving

Calories 260 Calories from Fat 120

	% Daily Value*
Total Fat 13g	20%
Saturated Fat 5g	25%
Cholesterol 30mg	10%
Sodium 660mg	28%
Total Carbohydrate 31g	10%
Dietary Fiber 0g	0%
Sugar 5g	
Protein 5g	

Vitamin A 4%	•	Vitamin C 2%
Calcium 15%	•	Iron 4%

* Percent daily values are based on a 2,000 calorie diet. Your daily values may be higher or lower depending on your calorie needs:

		Calories:	2,000	2,500
Total Fat	Less than		65g	80g
Sat Fat	Less than		20g	25g
Cholesterol	Less than		300mg	300mg
Sodium	Less than		2400mg	2400mg
Total Carbohydrate			300g	375g
Dietary Fiber			25g	30g

Calories per gram:
Fat 9 • Carbohydrate 4 • Protein 4

SERVINGS PER CONTAINER

The number of servings contained in the package.

TOTAL CARBOHYDRATE

The total grams of carbohydrate in one serving. The carbohydrate from dietary fibers and sugar is included, so don't count it twice.

Personal Food Plan

Your personal food plan shows the number of carbohydrate choices you need for each meal. Most adults need three to four choices at meals. You may need more or less. Your number of carbohydrate choices depends on your:

- age

- activity level

- gender

- weight goals

- eating preferences

- daily schedule

- diabetes medications

The table below shows the suggested carbohydrate choices per meal for women and men.

	TO LOSE WEIGHT	TO CONTROL WEIGHT	FOR THE VERY ACTIVE
Women	2–3 choices	3–4 choices	4–5 choices
Men	3–4 choices	4–5 choices	4–6 choices

Snacks may be included in your food plan. Snacks are usually one to two carbohydrate choices each. Some reasons for including snacks are:

- You're very hungry between meals or at mealtimes.

- You experience low blood glucose levels.

- You often overeat at meals.

- You're very active.

- Snacks are a regular part of your lifestyle.

- Your usual mealtimes are more than four to six hours apart.

Follow your food plan and test your blood glucose regularly. Keep accurate food and blood glucose records. This information helps you learn how to keep your blood glucose levels in target.

My Food Plan

Calories _____

Carbohydrate ___ gms (__%) Protein ___ gms (__%) Fat ___ gms (__%)

Breakfast Time: _8:00 am_

3-4   Carbohydrate Choices (or ___ starch ___fruit ___milk)

(45-60g)   2 toast   (2)

           ½ cup juice   (1)

0-1   Meat   1 oz Canadian bacon

1   Fat   1 tsp margarine

Physical Activity

It's hard to imagine anything better for you than physical activity. Even a small increase in physical activity can have a big effect on your diabetes and your health. It can:

- lower blood glucose levels

- help your body use insulin better

- create a feeling of health and well-being

- increase energy

- improve heart health and lower blood pressure

- increase strength, endurance, and flexibility

- lead to weight loss or maintenance

Physical activity doesn't have to be hard to be good. Simple things like walking, mowing the lawn, and house-work can help. The goal is to work up to thirty minutes of activity three times each week.

Your blood glucose level could go too low during exercise. Be sure to carry some form of carbohydrate with you during exercise in case this happens. (See page 36.)

Use the Activity Pyramid to decide on ways to include activity in your life. The best activity is the one you will do. Choose activities you enjoy.

The Activity Pyramid

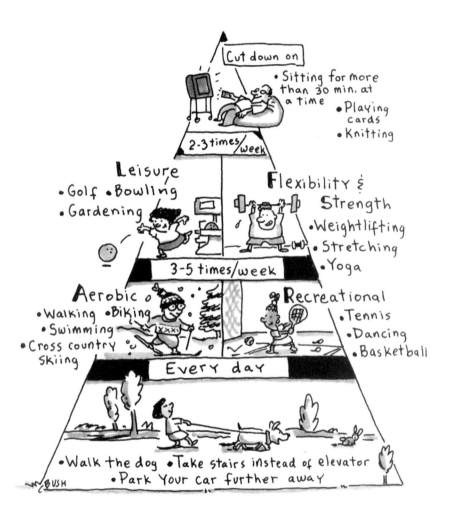

* If you have heart disease or other medical problems, talk to your doctor before starting a new activity.

Adapted from *The Activity Pyramid,* ©1996 Institute for Research and Education.

Until We Meet Again

- Test your blood glucose level every day at the proper testing times.

- Record the test results in your Diabetes Record Book.

- Complete your Food & Activity Record for at least three days before the next session.

- Stay active or become more active.

THE NEXT SESSION IS IN TWO WEEKS.

Day: _____

Date: _____

Time: _____

Place: _____

Bring the following:

- this book

- your completed Food & Activity Record

- your Diabetes Record Book with recorded test results

- your glucose meter, meter instruction manual, and test strips

- questions and experiences to share

Notes

Use this space to note questions, comments, and experiences
until the next session.

Welcome

In this session, you will:

- evaluate your self blood glucose test results

- learn how to take care of your blood glucose meter

- learn the causes, symptoms, and treatment for hypo-glycemia (low blood sugar) and hyperglycemia (high blood sugar)

- discover how fats, cholesterol, and alcohol affect diabetes control and healthy living

- develop personal action goals

- feel more confident about your ability to deal with your diabetes

Record Book Review

Your goal is to have at least one half (50%) of your blood glucose test results within the target range. If you reach this goal, your HbA_{1c} should be in target, too. Look back to page 14 to see what your HbA_{1c} target is.

Look at the test results you recorded in your Diabetes Record Book for the last two weeks. Fill in the blanks below.

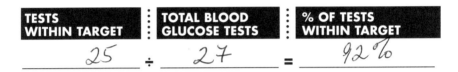

TESTS WITHIN TARGET		TOTAL BLOOD GLUCOSE TESTS		% OF TESTS WITHIN TARGET
25	÷	27	=	92 %

Divide the number of tests within target by the total number of tests. Are at least 50% (0.5 or higher) of your blood glucose tests within target? Check one.

☒ Yes. Change your testing schedule to three times a day, every three days.

☐ No. Continue testing three times a day, every day.

If you feel you can, commit to following the testing schedule given. Test at the following times every day you test:

• before breakfast

• before your main meal

• 1½ hours after your main meal

You may need a different testing schedule. If you do, your healthcare provider will discuss it with you.

Meter Maintenance and Quality Assurance

Your blood glucose test results help you and your healthcare provider make decisions about your treatment. It's important that they are accurate.

To assure accurate test results, your blood glucose meter needs a little upkeep. Follow the steps below to make sure it keeps working properly.

1. Clean your meter weekly, especially the movable parts.

2. Check your meter with control solution when opening a new vial of test strips. Check also if you get a result that doesn't seem right to you.

3. Be sure the code number on your meter matches the code number on your test strips.

4. If your meter has a calibration check strip, use it as directed.

If you have any questions about your meter, check with your healthcare provider. The customer service department of your meter manufacturer can help, too.

Blood Glucose Lows

It's normal for your blood glucose level to go up and down throughout the day. It goes up when you eat. It goes down as your body uses glucose for energy.

Sometimes your blood glucose level can go too low. Hypoglycemia, or low blood sugar, is defined as:

- a blood glucose level below 80 mg/dL plus symptoms

- any blood glucose level below 70 mg/dL

Learn how your body reacts to a low blood glucose level. Noticing symptoms early helps prevent further problems.

Symptoms of hypoglycemia include:

- feeling weak, dizzy, shaky, or sweaty

- pale, clammy skin

- fast heartbeat

- numb or tingling lips

- confusion

You can treat hypoglycemia yourself. Simply eat or drink something that contains 15 grams of carbohydrate. Treatment choices include:

- 3 glucose tablets

- $1/2$ cup fruit juice or regular soda pop

- 1 cup skim milk

- 6 to 7 hard candies

After about 15 minutes, your blood glucose level should go up. Then your symptoms will go away. You do not need to count food used to treat hypoglycemia as part of your food plan.

Untreated hypoglycemia can cause mood changes, poor coordination, and double vision. Be prepared. Keep a carbohydrate source handy at all times, especially in your car.

To prevent hypoglycemia, follow your food plan. Take your diabetes medication as prescribed.

CAUSES OF LOW BLOOD GLUCOSE

- eating less food than usual, particularly carbohydrate foods

- skipping or delaying a meal or snack

- getting more exercise than usual

- taking too much diabetes medication

Blood Glucose Highs

When you have diabetes, your blood glucose levels are higher than normal. If they go too high, it's called hyperglycemia. Symptoms of hyperglycemia include:

- feeling thirsty

- feeling tired

- going to the bathroom a lot

- blurry vision

Your treatment plan is aimed at keeping your blood glucose levels in target. Even so, your levels will sometimes be higher than your target range.

If your blood glucose level is too high too often, something needs to change. You may need to change your eating or activity habits. Sometimes you need a change in your treatment plan. You and your healthcare provider will decide what changes to make.

CAUSES OF HIGH BLOOD GLUCOSE

- eating more food than usual

- being less active than usual

- being under physical or emotional stress

- not taking enough diabetes medication

- being ill

Food Plan Review

It's a good idea to check in with yourself regularly about your eating habits. Most people have a mixture of successes and challenges with following a food plan. How is it going for you? Are you counting carbohydrates?

Take time to feel good about the things that are going well. You're doing a great job!

If you find that you are having difficulties, try to pinpoint problem areas. Think of ways to improve in these areas.

Be kind to yourself as you work on changing behaviors. Don't expect to do everything perfectly. But keep trying!

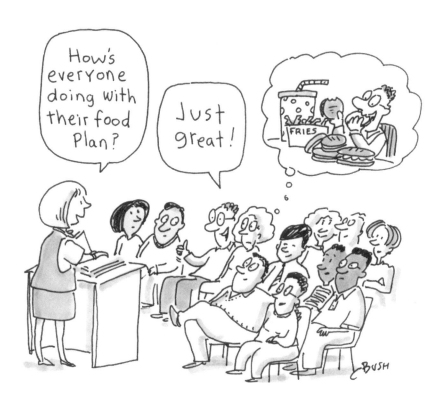

Keeping a Healthy Heart

Blood glucose control was the focus of learning about food and activity in Session 1. But food and activity also affect your heart health.

Heart health is important because diabetes increases your risk for heart disease. High cholesterol and high blood pressure add to your risk.

HEART ATTACKS PER 1000 PEOPLE

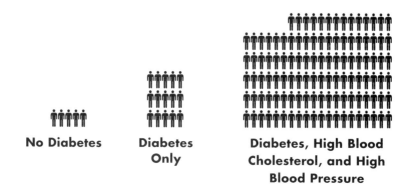

| No Diabetes | Diabetes Only | Diabetes, High Blood Cholesterol, and High Blood Pressure |

Everything you do to control your blood glucose levels also helps keep your heart healthy. Keeping your heart healthy helps improve your blood glucose control. It's a win-win situation. In addition, for a healthy heart:

• Don't smoke.

• Eat less fat, especially saturated fat.

• Become and stay physically active.

• Balance the stress in your life.

• Ask your provider about taking a low dose of aspirin.

ASSESSING YOUR HEART RISK

Check "Yes" if the statement is true, and check "No" if it is false.

Yes	No	
☐	☐	My HbA_{1c} is 7.5% or higher.*
☐	☐	My total cholesterol is 200 or higher.
☐	☐	My LDL cholesterol is 100 or higher.
☐	☐	My HDL cholesterol is under 40.
☐	☐	My triglyceride value is 200 or higher.
☐	☐	My blood pressure is 130/85 or higher.
☐	☐	I smoke.
☐	☐	I eat foods high in fat and high in saturated fat every day.
☐	☐	I eat less than five servings of fruit and/or vegetables a day.
☐	☐	I exercise less than three times a week.
☐	☐	I do not take a regular low dose of aspirin to help prevent heart disease.
☐	☐	One or more of my parents, brothers, or sisters has had a heart attack.
☐	☐	I have had a heart attack.
☐	☐	I have had a heart attack and have not discussed heart medications, including ACE inhibitors and beta blockers, with my doctor.
☐	☐	I am past menopause (women only).

Any "yes" answer means you are at risk for heart disease.
To reduce your risk, follow the suggestions on page 40.

* Based on 6% laboratory normal.

Cholesterol and Triglycerides

Healthy blood cholesterol and triglyceride levels are key to a healthy heart and blood vessels. Cholesterol is a waxy substance found in all body cells. Triglyceride is another name for fat.

Cholesterol and triglycerides are made in the body and are found in food. Most of the cholesterol we have is made in the body. Triglycerides come mostly from the food we eat.

Small packages called lipoproteins carry cholesterol and triglycerides through the bloodstream. There are two main lipoproteins:

• HDL (high-density lipoprotein)

• LDL (low-density lipoprotein)

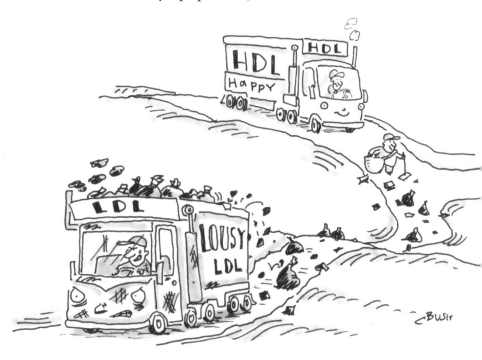

HDL carries cholesterol and triglycerides out of the blood. It's good to have high levels of HDL in your blood. Exercise and weight loss can increase HDL levels.

LDL deposits cholesterol and triglycerides, which can clog blood vessels. It's good to have low levels of LDL in your blood. Eating a healthy, low-fat diet lowers LDL levels. It also lowers triglyceride levels.

Total cholesterol is a combination of all the HDL and LDL in your blood.

You need to have your total cholesterol, triglycerides, HDL, and LDL checked regularly.

MEASURE	TARGETS
Total Cholesterol	Under 200 mg/dL (under 170 mg/dL optimal)
Triglycerides	Under 200 mg/dL (under 150 mg/dL optimal)
HDL	40 mg/dL or higher (45 mg/dL or higher optimal)
LDL	Under 100 mg/dL

Eating Less Fat

Carbohydrate is the body's first choice for energy. Fat is the second. Fat also provides essential fatty acids for normal body function.

There are two main kinds of fat in food. One is better for your heart than the other. But all fat is high in calories.

- Saturated fat is usually solid at room temperature. It raises blood cholesterol and is hard on your heart and blood vessels.

- Unsaturated fat is usually liquid at room temperature. It lowers blood cholesterol and is easier on your heart and blood vessels. Unsaturated fat can be polyunsaturated or monounsaturated.

SATURATED	POLYUNSATURATED	MONOUNSATURATED
Whole milk	Soybean oil	Olive oil
Meat	Safflower oil	Canola oil
Cheese	Corn oil	Avocados
Margarine, stick	Margarine, tub	Olives
Butter		Fish
Lard		
Shortening		

Most people eat too much fat. A healthy guideline is one to two fat servings (1 to 2 teaspoons) per meal. A fat serving can come from an actual fat, like margarine or oil, or from other foods. Examples of foods that have hidden added fat are potato chips and cookies.

Meat contains hidden fat, too. Try to eat no more than 5 to 8 ounces of cooked lean meat a day. If you have high cholesterol, try to eat less than 6 ounces a day. Six ounces of meat is about the size of two decks of cards.

Low-fat foods and low-fat cooking methods are good for your heart. Read the list of low-fat food choices. Is there one food in the list that you can substitute for a high-fat food you normally eat? Can you use low-fat cooking methods more often?

LOW-FAT FOOD CHOICES	LOW-FAT COOKING METHODS
Skim or 1% milk	Bake, broil, or grill meats
Light or nonfat sour cream	Use nonstick cookware for frying and baking
Light or nonfat cream cheese	Sauté in broth or wine
Low-fat or fat-free salad dressings	Try cooking spray instead of oil
Low-fat cheeses	Trim fat off meat before cooking
Fruits and vegetables	Remove skin from chicken and turkey
Steamed rice	Skip sauces, cream, gravy, and butter
Baked potatoes	
Low-fat or fat-free lunchmeats	
Chicken and turkey without skin	
Fish	
Lean cuts of beef or pork	

Diabetes and Alcohol

Alcohol is not converted into glucose. It is a source of calories, which the body must use as energy or store as fat. It can cause weight gain.

Alcohol lowers blood glucose levels. It can cause hypoglycemia, especially if you take a diabetes medication. The symptoms of hypoglycemia can appear to others as drunkenness. It's important to wear or carry medical identification at all times.

You can include alcohol in your food plan. Follow these simple guidelines.

- Use alcohol only when your diabetes is under control.

- Never drink alcohol on an empty stomach.

- Limit yourself to no more than two drinks per day.

- Wear a medical I.D. bracelet or necklace that says you have diabetes.

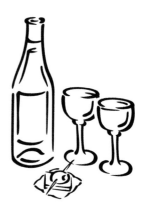

If you are taking any medications, ask your healthcare provider about alcohol. Avoid alcohol if:

- You are pregnant.

- You're trying to lose weight.

- You have high triglycerides.

- You have a history of alcohol or other drug abuse.

SERVING SIZES OF ALCOHOLIC DRINKS

- 12 ounces regular beer*

- 12 ounces light beer

- 4 ounces dry wine

- 12 ounces wine cooler*

- 1$^1/_2$ ounces scotch, whiskey, gin, etc.

- 2 ounces dry sherry

- $^1/_2$ ounce liqueur*

- 1 frozen margarita*

* Contains significant carbohydrate. (If you use fruit juice in a mixed drink, remember that juice contains carbohydrate. Also, be aware that alcohol adds calories.)

Setting Personal Goals

By now you know that staying healthy with diabetes means making some changes in your lifestyle. For example, you may need to:

- begin or do better at testing your blood glucose levels

- eat more healthfully

- become more physically active

- reduce stress

Setting a goal for yourself can help you make the changes you need to make. You know best what those changes are. An effective goal needs to be both reasonable and measurable.

SAMPLE GOALS

- I will test and record my blood glucose levels three times a day, every three days, for the next two weeks.

- Instead of one big meal, I will eat three small meals a day for one month.

- This week, I will ask my neighbor to be my regular walking partner.

A reasonable goal reflects your current health and abilities. It is something within your reach. A measurable goal is specific, not open-ended. It states what you will do and when you will do it.

A goal needs checkpoints for evaluating progress. A goal also deserves your commitment. Commitment turns something you feel you should do into something you believe you will do.

Think about what changes you want to make. Try to write a reasonable and measurable goal for yourself.

REASONABLE	UNREASONABLE
An inactive person writes, "I will walk for twenty minutes every Monday, Wednesday, and Thursday for the next three months."	An inactive person writes, "I will jog three miles five days a week."

MEASURABLE	NOT MEASURABLE
"I will drink 1% milk instead of whole milk for the next three months."	"I will eat better from now on."

Until We Meet Again

- Test your blood glucose level at the proper testing times.

- Record the test results in your Diabetes Record Book.

- Complete your Food & Activity Record for at least three of the days you test.

- Work on the goal(s) you set for yourself.

THE NEXT SESSION IS:

Day:

Date:

Time:

Place:

Bring the following:

- this book

- your completed Food & Activity Record

- your Diabetes Record Book with recorded test results

- your My Personal Goals Action Plan

- your glucose meter, meter instruction manual, and test strips

- questions and experiences to share

Notes

Use this space to note questions, comments, and experiences until the next session.

Welcome

In this session, you will:

- understand how blood glucose numbers relate to your HbA$_{1c}$ value

- learn problem-solving techniques for times when blood glucose numbers are out of target range

- learn how illness affects blood glucose numbers and what to do when you're ill

- recognize the importance of foot care and learn how to care for your feet

- discover tips for following your food plan at restaurants, parties, and special events

- learn how to estimate portion sizes

- feel affirmed in your efforts to manage your diabetes

Blood Glucose Numbers and HbA$_{1c}$

Your HbA$_{1c}$ value represents your average blood glucose level over the past two months. If you haven't had an HbA$_{1c}$ test yet, ask your healthcare provider to do one.

Your HbA$_{1c}$ value needs to be no more than 1 to 1.5 percentage points over normal. Look back to page 14 to see what your HbA$_{1c}$ target is.

The goal is to get your HbA$_{1c}$ value in target and keep it there. Your value can be in target, even when some blood glucose numbers are out of target.

Some of your blood glucose numbers will be out of target. That's okay. Your goal is to have at least one half of them (50%) within range. When you reach this goal, your HbA$_{1c}$ should be in target too.

Look at the test results you recorded in your Diabetes Record Book since the last session. Fill in the blanks below.

TESTS WITHIN TARGET	TOTAL BLOOD GLUCOSE TESTS	% OF TESTS WITHIN TARGET

_____ ÷ _____ = _____

Divide the number of tests within target by the total number of tests. Are at least 50% (0.5 or higher) of your blood glucose tests within target? Check one.

☐ Yes. Change your testing schedule to three times a day, every three days.

☐ No. Continue testing three times a day, every day.

If you feel you can, commit to following the testing schedule given. Test at the following times every day you test:

• before breakfast

• before your main meal

• 1½ hours after your main meal

You may need a different testing schedule. If you do, your healthcare provider will discuss it with you.

Using Your Blood Glucose Numbers

You need to pay attention when your blood glucose numbers are out of target. Often you can figure out why it's happening.

Let's look at an example. Suppose you have a high blood glucose level before dinner. Ask yourself what might have caused it. Maybe you ate a big lunch that day. Maybe you missed your usual afternoon exercise.

When you figure out why your blood glucose level is high, then you can make changes to prevent it from happening again. The causes of high blood glucose are listed on page 38.

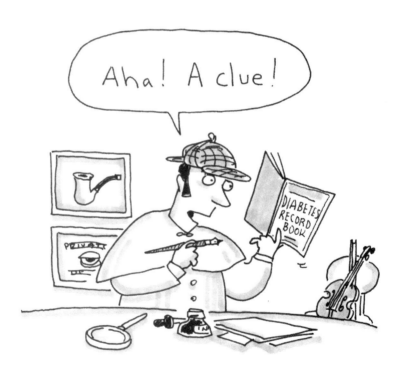

Write notes in your Diabetes Record Book that might help you understand your numbers. Special events, like a holiday meal, can cause a high level. So can other changes in your usual eating and activity schedules. Examples include parties, vacations, restaurant meals, and illness.

Sometimes you have a high blood glucose level that you can't explain. Follow these steps to get more information.

1. Retest immediately—the first reading might have been a mistake.

2. Check meter accuracy—the meter may not be working properly.

3. Test before meals for the next couple of days—you may notice a pattern of high levels. If you notice a pattern, call your healthcare provider.

Sick Day Management

An illness, like a cold or the flu, can cause high blood glucose levels. High levels can appear even before the symptoms of illness do.

You need to pay special attention to your diabetes during an illness. This includes testing your blood glucose more often than usual.

You also need to keep eating, even when you aren't feeling well. You need to eat small amounts of carbohydrate foods. This is especially important if you take a diabetes medication. Carbohydrate foods give your body energy to heal and help control your blood glucose levels. It's okay to sip regular soda pop or have sweetened jello when you're sick. Sometimes these are the only carbohydrate foods that will stay down.

REASONS TO CALL YOUR HEALTHCARE PROVIDER

- Most of your blood glucose test results are over 240 mg/dL for three days in a row.

- Your blood glucose level falls below 70 mg/dL and you have symptoms of hypoglycemia.

- You have vomiting or diarrhea that lasts longer than six hours.

- You can't keep liquids down.

Here are some important things to do when you are ill:

- If you take a diabetes medication, continue the usual dose. Your healthcare provider will tell you if it needs to be changed.

- Check and record your blood glucose level every two to four hours.

- Try to have one carbohydrate choice (15 grams carbohydrate) for each hour that you are awake.

- Drink plenty of sugar-free liquids to replace body fluids lost during illness. Examples include water, broth, and tea. Sip liquids slowly.

CARBOHYDRATE CHOICES FOR SICK DAYS

- 1/2 cup regular soda pop
- 6 saltine crackers
- 1/2 cup fruit juice
- 1 slice dry toast
- 1 cup soup (not broth)
- 1/2 cup regular (sweetened) gelatin
- 1/2 cup cooked cereal
- 1 popsicle (60 to 80 calories)
- 1/2 cup ice cream or frozen yogurt
- 1 tablespoon honey or sugar
- 1/4 cup sherbet or fruit ice

Blood Pressure

Diabetes can affect the heart and circulation, the eyes, the kidneys, and the nerves. Your healthcare provider will check the health of these organs and systems as part of your regular diabetes care.

One thing that needs to be checked is your blood pressure. High blood pressure puts extra strain on the heart. It also can damage small blood vessels in the eyes and kidneys. It adds to the risk for heart, eye, and kidney problems.

Blood pressure is recorded as two numbers. The upper number is the systolic blood pressure—the pressure when your heart is contracting. The lower number is the diastolic pressure—the pressure when your heart is relaxed. If either number is high, your risk for heart disease is increased.

The recommended blood pressure for people with diabetes is 130/85 or less. This is a little lower than for the general population. Make sure your blood pressure is checked at every healthcare visit.

Regular exercise can help you lower blood pressure. Using less salt (sodium) and moderate weight loss also can help. Sometimes medication is needed to lower blood pressure to a safe level.

Stress can contribute to the development of high blood pressure. Take steps to balance stress in your life. Set aside time each day to read, take a walk, or do something you enjoy. Relaxation or meditation classes also may help.

Talk to your healthcare provider about your blood pressure and how to control it.

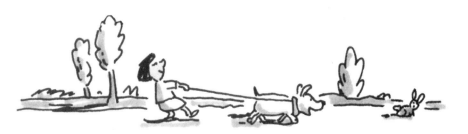

Five Steps to Healthy Feet

One more reason to keep your blood glucose levels in target is your feet. That may sound funny, but think about it. High blood glucose levels affect your heart and circulation. Where's the farthest your blood has to travel in your body? Your feet!

Poor circulation and nerve damage usually affect the feet and lower legs first. You might feel numbness, tingling, or pain. You might have sores that won't heal.

These problems can become very serious. You need to take care of your feet every day to prevent this from happening. Follow the five steps for healthy feet on the next page.

FOOT-CARE DON'TS

- Don't go barefoot.
- Don't soak your feet.
- Don't use chemical treatments, sharp instruments, sandpaper, or pumice to treat calluses, corns, or other foot problems.
- Don't expose your feet to extreme heat or cold.
- Don't put heating pads or hot water bottles on your feet.
- Don't sit with your legs crossed.
- Don't try to break in a new pair of shoes by wearing them for a whole day.

Step 1: Keep your blood glucose levels in target. We've already said a lot about this. The best way to stay healthy and prevent problems is to control blood glucose levels.

Step 2: Practice good foot-care habits. Wash your feet with mild soap and water every day. Dry them completely. Trim toenails straight across; use lotion if your skin is dry. Wear socks and shoes made from natural materials such as cotton, wool, or leather. Make sure your toes have room to wiggle in your shoes.

Step 3: Check your feet daily. Look them over thoroughly—top, bottom, and between your toes. Use a mirror to check hard-to-see places. Look for corns and calluses, ingrown nails, cuts, blisters, or cracked skin. If you notice any sign of infection, call your healthcare provider. Signs of infection include redness, red streaks, swelling, oozing, warm spots, and pain.

Step 4: Treat foot injuries immediately. Minor blisters, cuts, or scrapes can be cleaned and treated with antibiotic cream. Check daily to make sure the area is healing. Stay alert for signs of infection. If you're unsure how to treat a foot injury, call your healthcare provider.

Step 5: Visit your healthcare provider every three to four months. Remove your shoes and socks to ensure that your feet are examined at every visit. Discuss any problems or questions you have. Ask if you need and qualify for prescription footwear.

Food Planning: Keys to Success

From feet to food! Diabetes truly affects every part of your life. That's why it's so important for you to learn about diabetes and food planning. The more you know, the more successful you'll be at living well with diabetes.

Two important keys to success in food planning are:

• making healthy food choices

• choosing portions that fit your food plan

Once you learn these skills, you can eat anywhere with confidence. You will know how to follow your food plan in any situation.

For you, making healthy food choices includes paying attention to *carbohydrate* and *fat.* You need to count carbohydrates. This helps keep your blood glucose levels in target. And, whenever possible, you need to choose carbohydrate and other foods that are low in fat. This helps keep your heart healthy.

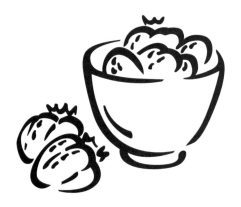

Eating the *right amount* of these foods is the next challenge. Though you may measure out servings at first, you won't always be able to. Instead you need to learn to estimate portions by sight.

Practice estimating portions. Learn what $\frac{1}{2}$ cup of mashed potatoes looks like on a dinner plate. Put the same amount in a bowl. Weigh out a 3-ounce baked potato and a 3-ounce boneless chicken breast.

After awhile you'll be able to dish up a single serving every time without measuring. But check yourself once in awhile. When you're estimating portions, they tend to grow over time.

FOOD AND AMOUNT		SERVING-SIZE SHORTCUT
3 ounces meat	=	deck of playing cards
$\frac{1}{2}$ cup ice cream	=	tennis ball
1 ounce cheese	=	4 stacked dice
1 teaspoon butter or margarine	=	1 pat
$\frac{1}{2}$ cup mashed potatoes	=	tennis ball
1 3-ounce baked potato	=	2 whole eggs

Strategies for Dining Out

Eating at a restaurant used to be a luxury. Today most of us eat out regularly. Diabetes doesn't change this.

You can enjoy eating away from home and still take care of your diabetes. Carbohydrate counting, making healthy food choices, and portion control are important. So is planning.

If you eat out often, select foods and portions that equal the carbohydrate choices in your food plan. Your skill at estimating portion sizes will help here. Unfortunately, you can't "save" carbohydrates from one meal and have them at another. Try to follow your food plan for the meal you're eating out.

If it's a special occasion, maybe you can indulge a little. Extra exercise can help make up for a splurge once in a while.

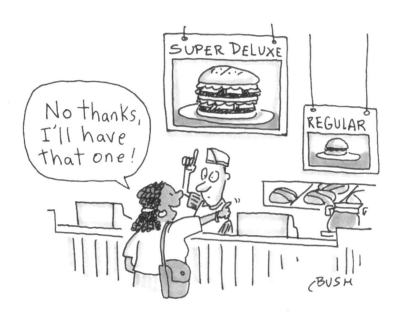

The chart on pages 94–95 shows the carbohydrate choices for some popular restaurant menu items. Smart, lower-fat choices are marked with a ♥. Use the chart and the guidelines below to dine out healthfully.

Watch the fat. Restaurant food often has a lot of added fat. Look for broiled, baked, grilled, or steamed menu items. Remove skin from poultry and trim fat from meat. It's okay to save up fat servings to use for a special meal.

Eat moderate portions. Restaurant portions are usually large. Learn to estimate appropriate serving sizes. Avoid menu items described as "super" or "deluxe." Share, leave food on your plate, or ask for a doggy bag.

Ask for what you want. Request that food be prepared with less fat. Get salad dressing "on the side," and butter your own potato. You'll probably use less if you add it yourself. Try substituting a salad or a baked potato for French fries.

Enjoy yourself! If you overindulge, don't panic. Instead, go for a walk or go dancing. If you find that you overeat often, try to plan ahead. Develop strategies for avoiding temptation, such as having a salad before a pizza meal.

Personal Goals Checkpoint

Remember the goal you wrote on My Personal Goals Action Plan at the last session? Do you think you accomplished it?

If you've done well on your goal, think about what has helped you. Commit to continuing your healthy behaviors. And congratulate yourself! Then if you're ready, write another goal to work on. Look back on page 48 to review how to write a goal.

If you haven't done so well, ask yourself why. Try to identify obstacles. Then you can work on ways to overcome them. Look at your goal again. Did you set it too high? Make sure it is something you feel you can do. If it isn't, you may need to rewrite it.

Be kind to yourself as you try to make changes. It took a long time to develop your current behaviors. Making a change that will last can take awhile.

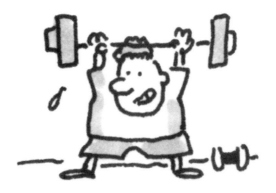

Until We Meet Again

- Test your blood glucose level at the proper testing times.

- Record the test results in your Diabetes Record Book.

- Complete your Food & Activity Record for at least three of the days you test.

- Work on the goal(s) you set for yourself.

THE NEXT SESSION IS:

Day:

Date:

Time:

Place:

Bring the following:

- this book

- your completed Food & Activity Record

- your Diabetes Record Book with recorded test results

- your My Personal Goals Action Plan

- your glucose meter, meter instruction manual, and test strips

- questions and experiences to share

Notes

Use this space to note questions, comments, and experiences until the next session.

Welcome

In this session, you will:

• learn how stress affects blood glucose levels and develop strategies for balancing stress

• learn how diabetes changes over time and how this affects treatment

• understand why regular diabetes care visits are important and what to expect from your healthcare provider

• learn simple eating tips that can help control blood glucose levels, improve nutrition, and enhance health

• understand the need for continuing diabetes education

• better appreciate your ability to self-manage your diabetes

Keeping Blood Glucose Levels in Target

You've probably made a lot of changes in your life over the past several months. You're testing your blood glucose. You may eat differently than before. You may be more active than you were three months ago.

You're making changes to help keep your blood glucose levels in target. If they're in target at least half the time, good for you! Celebrate your success and keep it up! If they're not, you need to figure out why and do something about it.

The most important thing to do is to follow your treatment plan. Even when you do, your blood glucose levels can be out of target. This can happen when there is:

- a crisis or change in your life that upsets your schedule or causes stress

- a change in your diabetes

Look at the test results you recorded in your Diabetes Record Book since the last session. Fill in the blanks below.

TESTS WITHIN TARGET	**TOTAL BLOOD GLUCOSE TESTS**	**% OF TESTS WITHIN TARGET**

_____ ÷ _____ = _____

Divide the number of tests within target by the total number of tests. Are at least 50% (0.5 or higher) of your blood glucose tests within target? Check one.

☐ Yes. Change your testing schedule to three times a day, every three days.

☐ No. Continue testing three times a day, every day.

If you feel you can, commit to following the testing schedule given. Test at the following times every day you test:

• before breakfast

• before your main meal

• 1½ hours after your main meal

You may need a different testing schedule. If you do, your healthcare provider will discuss it with you.

Balancing Stress

Stress can make blood glucose levels hard to control. Both negative and positive events can cause stress. Illness, moving, marriage, retirement—all are stressful.

Stress also can interfere with your diabetes care schedule. Then it's even harder to keep blood glucose levels in target. And that causes more stress!

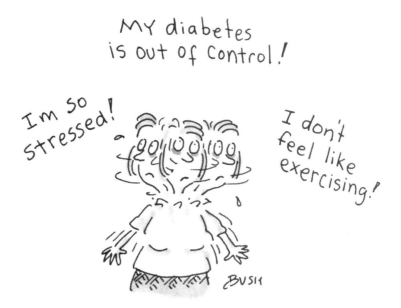

The Balancing Stress Pyramid shows ways to keep your life balanced. Decide what works for you. And always follow your treatment plan, especially during stressful times.

Balancing Stress Pyramid

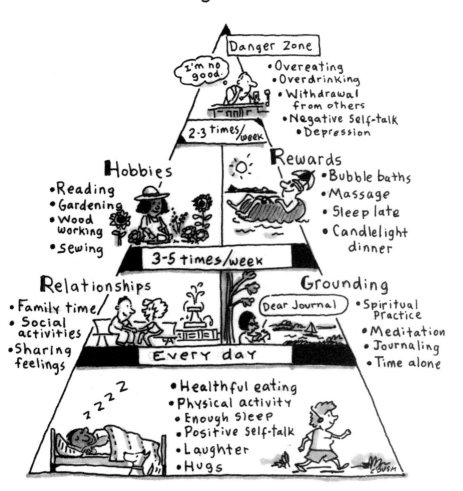

The Natural Changes of Diabetes

Over time, diabetes causes changes in the body's cells and in the pancreas. These are natural changes that happen when you have diabetes. The changes happen at different times for different people. Generally they develop over a number of years.

These changes cause two things to happen:

• The body's cells become resistant to the action of insulin.

• The pancreas first makes more insulin then eventually makes less and less.

As these changes happen, your treatment plan needs to change, too. You may need to add a medication or change your medication. Which medication you need depends on what changes are taking place.

The graph below shows how diabetes develops and progresses. Each stage is numbered and explained on the next page. Understanding these changes will help you understand your treatment. If you have questions, be sure to ask your healthcare provider.

HOW DIABETES DEVELOPS AND CHANGES OVER TIME

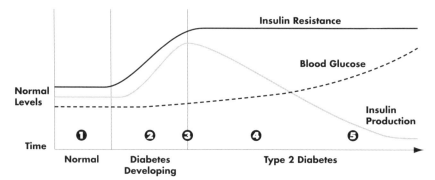

1 Before diabetes is diagnosed, the pancreas produces the right amount of insulin. The body's cells use the insulin properly. This keeps blood glucose levels normal.

2 The body's cells become resistant to insulin. The pancreas works hard to make more insulin to overcome the resistance. Blood glucose levels go above normal but not high enough to be diabetes (impaired fasting glucose or impaired glucose tolerance). People in this stage are at risk for developing diabetes. Exercise and healthy eating may help prevent or delay the onset of diabetes.

3 The pancreas can't make enough insulin. Blood glucose levels go higher still. Though diabetes can be detected by blood tests at this stage, it often isn't for several years. When diabetes is diagnosed, a food plan and activity are prescribed. Also, a diabetes pill might be prescribed either to reduce insulin resistance or to increase insulin production. (See the table of diabetes pills on pages 90–91.)

4 Insulin resistance continues to be a problem and insulin production continues to drop off. Both problems need to be treated in this stage. A combination of two different pills— one to treat each problem—is generally prescribed.

5 The pancreas eventually may make very little insulin. When insulin production drops too low, diabetes pills alone just aren't enough to treat the problem. At this point, insulin injections are needed. A diabetes pill that treats insulin resistance may be used along with insulin injections.

Staying Healthy for a Lifetime

Because diabetes changes over time, you need to see your healthcare provider regularly. You and your provider will review your blood glucose records and laboratory test results. You will discuss your treatment plan and any changes that may be needed.

You need to visit your healthcare provider every three to four months. The Physical Tune-up on pages 96–97 is a one-year schedule for keeping track of your visits. It shows all the tests and exams you should expect to have and the target for each. If you have questions about your care, be sure to ask your provider.

Regular diabetes care visits help you stay in control of your diabetes and your blood glucose levels. Research has shown that blood glucose control helps prevent diabetes complications.

BLOOD GLUCOSE CONTROL REDUCES THE RISK OF...	BY...
Eye disease	76%
Heart problems	42%
Kidney disease	56%
Nerve damage	60%

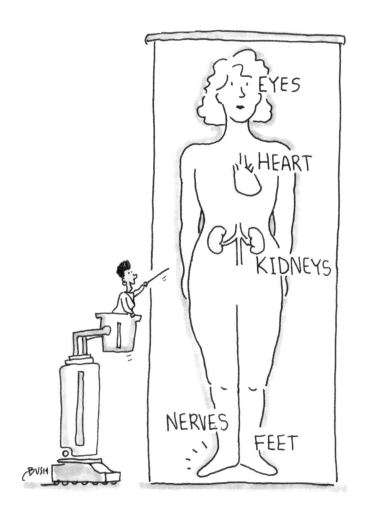

You are your own primary care giver. You take care of your diabetes every day. Following your treatment plan and keeping track of your blood glucose levels will help you stay healthy.

The Food Pyramid

By now you're an expert at carbohydrate counting. You know the importance of spacing carbohydrates out over the day. You also know that reducing fat in your diet is healthy for you and for your heart.

But like everyone else, it's important for you to include a variety of foods in your diet. This helps you get all the nutrients you need for good health. It also helps prevent "food boredom," which can lead to unhealthy eating behaviors.

The Food Pyramid is an excellent guide to healthful eating. It shows foods divided into six groups. It also tells you the number of servings needed from each group every day for good nutrition.

The carbohydrate food groups are light gray in the pyramid. Many healthy and delicious foods are carbohydrate foods. Be sure to include them in your meals. Just don't forget to count them!

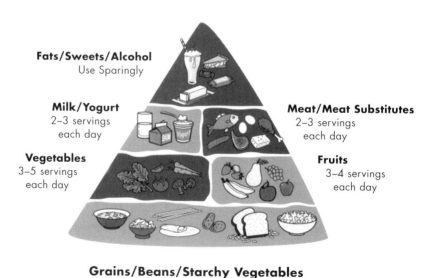

Fats/Sweets/Alcohol
Use Sparingly

Milk/Yogurt
2–3 servings
each day

Meat/Meat Substitutes
2–3 servings
each day

Vegetables
3–5 servings
each day

Fruits
3–4 servings
each day

Grains/Beans/Starchy Vegetables
6 or more servings each day

Five Good Food Habits

The Five Good Food Habits are simple ways to put the food pyramid to work. They are "helpful hints" to help you stick with your food plan, control your blood glucose levels, and stay healthy. Sample menus based on the habits are on pages 98–100.

Good Food Habit 1: Choose a variety of healthful foods. Variety helps you stick with your food plan, enjoy your meals and snacks, and get the energy and nutrition you need each day.

- Involve all your senses when you eat. Food should look good, smell good, feel good, taste good, and even sound good.

- Choose foods from every area of the food pyramid each day.

- Consider the colors of foods when planning meals. Strive for variety and balance.

- Try an exotic fruit or something else totally new.

- Mix and match different vegetables for interesting salads.

- Walk the aisles of the grocery store to become aware of all the foods available. (But not when you're hungry!)

- Try a new recipe once a week.

Good Food Habit 2: Eat moderate amounts. You can eat almost any food, if you watch portions. And you may see an added benefit—weight loss. A loss of just ten to twenty pounds can help improve blood glucose levels.

- Practice measuring. Learn how to "eyeball" portions.

- Try leaving serving bowls off the table to avoid second helpings.

- Sit, slow down, and enjoy. Fast eaters tend to eat more.

- Add high-fiber, low-calorie foods like raw vegetables to fill you up.

- Try putting your fork down between bites.

Good Food Habit 3: Choose low-fat foods often. There are many options for enjoying the foods you like without eating too much fat. Make gradual changes that will last a lifetime. This can help you reach weight or cholesterol goals.

- Substitute plain nonfat yogurt for mayonnaise or sour cream.

- Choose chicken, lean beef, or fish.

- Bake, broil, steam, or grill instead of frying.

- Look for snacks with fewer than 3 grams of fat per serving.

- Choose nonfat or low-fat dairy foods when possible.

- Try smaller portions, or low-fat versions, of high-fat foods.

- Try using one-third to one-half less fat or oil in recipes.

Good Food Habit 4: Eat at regular times. Eating small, frequent meals and snacks gives your body the energy it needs. It also spreads the carbohydrate "workload" out, so your pancreas doesn't get overloaded.

- Don't forget to eat breakfast. It helps to keep quick, convenient breakfast foods available.

- Try not to skip meals.

- Build in a snack to help control portions at the next meal.

- Plan your snacks and keep them handy.

- Wait two hours after a meal before having a snack.

Good Food Habit 5: Stay physically active. This isn't exactly a food habit, but it's very important. Physical activity can help lower your blood glucose levels. It also can help you lose weight and lower your cholesterol.

- Look for activities you enjoy and vary your workouts.

- Strive for consistency. Once you start, keep it up!

- Make an appointment with yourself to exercise.

- Ask a friend to join you or listen to music.

- Exercise at a pace that allows you to talk comfortably. Panting is not aerobic.

- Start with five to ten minutes of exercise and build up to at least thirty minutes per session.

Staying in Charge of Diabetes

By now you know that you need to care for your diabetes every day. And the more you know and understand about diabetes, the better you'll be able to manage it.

You've already learned a lot about diabetes and how to stay healthy. As time goes on, you will continue to learn and to increase your self-care skills.

Be sure to learn about the many opportunities for continuing diabetes education and support in your community. Your healthcare provider can help you identify classes, books, support groups, and other learning resources. There is also a resource list on pages 101–104 of this book.

Remember, too, that your family and friends can be your strongest support system. Include them in your learning process, and share your experience of living with diabetes with them.

Personal Goals Checkpoint

It's time to check in with your personal goals. How do you think you're doing?

If you're doing well, congratulate yourself! Commit to continuing your healthy behaviors. Then if you're ready, write another goal to work on. Look back on page 48 to review how to write a goal.

If you're struggling, try to identify your obstacles. Then you can work on ways to overcome them. If needed, rewrite your goal to reflect your current desires and ability.

Remember you are making changes that are meant to last a lifetime. Be patient, and keep up the good work!

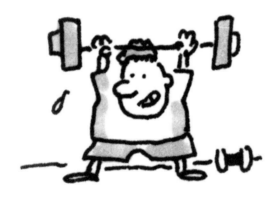

Congratulations!

This is to certify that

_____

Name

completed the program

Type 2 Diabetes

BASICS

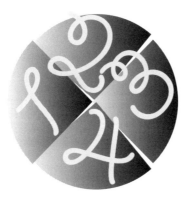

_____   _____

Educator   Date

APPENDIX

Diabetes Pills Used to Treat Type 2 Diabetes

SULFONYLUREAS (SULFA-BASED) SECOND GENERATION

Stimulate the pancreas to release more insulin.

Generic Name/ Trade Name	Common Starting Dose	Maximum Dose per Day	Schedule for Taking
Glyburide/ DiaBeta®	1.25–5 mg	20 mg	1–2 times daily with meals
Glyburide/ Micronase®	1.25–5 mg	20 mg	1–2 times daily with meals
Glyburide/ Glynase®	1.50–3 mg	12 mg	1–2 times daily with meals
Glipizide/ Glucotrol®	5 mg	40 mg	1–2 times daily, ¹/₂ hour before meals
Glipizide/ Glucotrol XL™ (extended release)	2.50–5 mg	20 mg	1 time daily with meal
Glimepiride/ Amaryl®	1–2 mg	8 mg	1 time daily with meal

BIGUANIDES

Decrease the release of glucose by the liver and make the cells more sensitive to insulin.

Generic Name/ Trade Name	Common Starting Dose	Maximum Dose per Day	Schedule for Taking
Metformin/ Glucophage®	500– 1000 mg	2550 mg	1–3 times daily with meals

New medications and formulations are approved by the Food and Drug Administration on an ongoing basis. Ask your healthcare provider for the latest information.

90

THIAZOLIDINEDIONES

Make the cells more sensitive to insulin and decrease the release of glucose by the liver.

Generic Name/ Trade Name	Common Starting Dose	Maximum Dose per Day	Schedule for Taking
Rosiglitazone/ Avandia®	4 mg	8 mg	1-2 times daily with meals
Pioglitazone/ Actos®	15-30 mg	45 mg	1 time daily

MEGLITINIDES

Stimulate the pancreas to release insulin over a shorter period of time (after meals).

Generic Name/ Trade Name	Common Starting Dose	Maximum Dose per Day	Schedule for Taking
Repaglinide/ Prandin®	0.5-1 mg	16 mg	2-4 times daily with meals

ALPHA GLUCOSIDASE INHIBITORS

Slow the body's absorption of carbohydrates.

Generic Name/ Trade Name	Common Starting Dose	Maximum Dose per Day	Schedule for Taking
Acarbose/ Precose®	25 mg	300 mg	3 times daily with meals
Miglitol/ Glyset®	25 mg	300 mg	3 times daily with meals

Diabetes Supply Shopping List

Your healthcare provider will help you fill out this list.

Date _____

Blood glucose meter _____

Test strips _____

Lancet device _____

Lancets _____

Insulin (if applicable) _____

Syringes (if applicable) _____

Sharps container _____

Treatment for reactions _____

Medical identification _____

Ketone testing _____

Suppliers_____

_____

_____

Other_____

_____

_____

_____

_____

Disposal of Household Sharps

Needles (syringes) and lancets need to be disposed of properly to make sure others are not injured. To dispose of needles and lancets:

- Place used sharps (needles and lancets) in a puncture-resistant container that can be secured with a cap or lid. Plastic detergent or soda bottles with screw caps work well. The Environmental Protection Agency has conducted studies showing that two-liter plastic soda bottles withstand the solid waste disposal process and compacting better than other containers.

- Label the container "Home Sharps" or "Household Sharps." If your area offers curb-side recycling, indicate that the sharps container should not be recycled by labeling it "Do Not Recycle."

- It's usually a good idea to inform your trash collector that your trash will include a container with household sharps. The container may need to be separated from the other garbage.

Dining Out Favorites

If you count fat grams, women should aim for no more than 20-25 grams of fat per meal, and men should aim for no more than 25-35 grams. For side dishes or snacks, try to keep below 3 grams of fat per carbohydrate serving.

FAST FOOD	CARBOHYDRATE CHOICES
♥ Baked potato, plain, (Wendy's) 5	
Big Fish Sandwich® (Burger King) 4	
Burger, large (Burger King Whopper®) 3	
♥ Burger, small 2	
Chicken breast, original (KFC) 1	
Chicken burrito (Taco Bell) 3	
Chicken McNuggets®, 6 (McDonald's) 1	
♥ Chili, 12 ounces (Wendy's) 2	
French fries, small 2	
Onion rings, small . . . . 2$^1/_2$	
Personal Pan Pizza®, pepperoni (Pizza Hut) 5	
♥ Roast beef, regular (Arby's) 2	
♥ Santa Fe Turkey Sandwich (Bruegger's) 4	
♥ Turkey breast, 6" (Subway) 3	

MEXICAN

♥ Taco, 7" soft-shell 1
Beef enchilada, 6" 2
Burrito de frijole (bean), 9" 4
Chimichanga, 6 ounces 3
Nachos, with beef and beans, 6 to 8 . . . . 3$^1/_2$
Taco salad, large 4
Taco, large, fried tortilla, sour cream 3
Quesadilla 2

♥ Smart choices for heart health or weight loss

94

	CARBOHYDRATE
INDIAN	**CHOICES**
❤ Chapati, 6"	1
❤ Naan, 1 small loaf	1
❤ Basmati rice, $^1/_2$ cup	1
Samosa, lamb-filled	1
❤ Dal (dhal), $^1/_2$ cup	1

ASIAN

❤ Chicken and vegetables, 2 cups	2
Egg roll, 1 small	1
❤ Chow mein, 2 cups	2
Rice, fried, and meat, 1 cup	2
Sweet and sour pork, $1^1/_2$ cups	4
❤ Rice, white, 1 cup	3
❤ Wonton soup, 1 cup with 2 wontons	1

ITALIAN

Cannelloni, 4 stuffed noodles	2
❤ Chicken cacciatore, 1/2 breast	1
Fettuccini primavera, $1^1/_2$ cups	2
❤ Lasagna, beef 3" by 4"	1
Manicotti, cheese with sauce, 2	3
❤ Marinara sauce, $^1/_2$ cup	1

DESSERT AND SPECIALITY ITEMS

Bismark (Dunkin Donuts)	3
Blueberry muffin (Arby's)	2
❤ Cafe Latte, tall, nonfat milk (Starbucks)	1
Cake, 2" square with frosting	2
Cinnamon crisps (Taco Bell)	2
Glazed Donut (Dunkin Donuts)	$1^1/_2$
❤ Honey-grain Bagel (Bruegger's)	4
Sugar-free apple pie, $^1/_6$ pie (Perkins)	4
❤ Sugar-free yogurt, $^1/_2$ cup (TCBY)	1
❤ Vanilla cone, small (McDonald's)	$1^1/_2$

❤ Smart choices for heart health or weight loss

95

Physical Tune-up

You need to see your healthcare provider at least two to four times per year.

Check Points	Target	Initial Checkup Date:
Height		
Weight		
Blood Pressure	Under 130/85	
HbA$_{1c}$	Optimal: Less than 1.0 over lab normal Desirable: 1.5 or less over lab normal	
Alb/Cr Ratio	Under 30 mg/G	
Total Cholesterol	Optimal: Under 170 mg/dL Desirable: Under 200 mg/dL	
HDL	Optimal: 45 mg/dL or higher Desirable: 40 mg/dL or higher	
Chol/HDL Ratio	4.5 or under	
LDL	Under 100 mg/dL	
Triglycerides	Optimal: Under 150 mg/dL Desirable: Under 200 mg/dL	
EKG (electrocardiogram)	Normal	
Thyroid Function (TSH)	0.2-5.5 µIU/mL (may vary by lab)	
Dental Exam		
Eye Exam (dilated pupil)		
Foot Exam		
Meter Check		
Observed Injection (if taking insulin)		

Target ranges for elderly may vary, so check with your healthcare provider.
©2000 International Diabetes Center, Institute for Research and Education.

3 Month Visit	6 Month Visit	9 Month Visit	One Year Visit
Date:	Date:	Date:	Date:

Sample Menus*

MENUS FOR WOMEN WHO WANT TO LOSE WEIGHT

About 1200 calories

BREAKFAST

1 slice whole wheat toast

1 teaspoons margarine

$^1/_3$ melon

Coffee

BREAKFAST

Vegetable omelet ($^1/_2$ cup egg substitute, vegetables)

1 slice toast

1 teaspoon margarine

2 small plums

LUNCH

Chicken vegetable soup

Sandwich (2 slices whole wheat bread, 2 ounces water-packed tuna, and 1 tablespoon fat-free or light salad dressing)

1 orange

Diet soda pop

LUNCH

1 cup spaghetti with $^1/_2$ cup tomato sauce

Tossed salad with 2 tablespoons fat-free or light salad dressing

$^1/_2$ cup sliced peaches

Coffee

DINNER

3 ounces grilled fish

1 small baked potato

1 cup broccoli

1 tablespoon low-fat sour cream

1 cup skim milk

DINNER

1 low-calorie frozen dinner

1 cup green beans

Iced tea

SNACK IDEAS (CHOOSE ONE)

1 piece fresh fruit

1 ounce fat-free tortilla chips (about 12 chips)

$^1/_3$ cup frozen yogurt

Frozen juice bar

3 cups air-popped popcorn

---

*The menus on pages 98–100 are reprinted from *Five Good Food Habits*, ©1995 International Diabetes Center.

MENUS FOR MEN WHO WANT TO LOSE WEIGHT OR WOMEN WHO WANT TO MAINTAIN WEIGHT

About 1500 calories

BREAKFAST

1 English muffin

1 teaspoon margarine

4 ounces orange juice

Sugar-free jam

Tea

BREAKFAST

1 cup oatmeal

1 cup 1% milk

1 small banana

Coffee

LUNCH

Sandwich (2 slices bread, 1 ounce ham, 1 ounce low-fat cheese, mustard)

1 cup low-fat cabbage salad

1 apple

Iced tea

LUNCH

1 cup chili

6 saltine crackers

1 ounce low-fat cheese

Sugar-free gelatin

1 cup melon

Carrot and celery sticks

Sugar-free lemonade

DINNER

$1^1/_2$ cups casserole (3 ounces turkey, pasta, vegetables, low-fat cream soup)

Tossed salad with 2 tablespoons fat-free or light salad dressing

Sugar-free gelatin

1 cup 1% or skim milk

DINNER

2 pieces vegetable pizza

Vegetable sticks

1 piece fresh fruit

Diet soda pop

SNACK IDEAS (CHOOSE ONE)

2 ounces pretzels

2 low-fat cookies, 1 cup skim milk

1 piece fresh fruit

MENUS FOR MEN WHO WANT TO MAINTAIN WEIGHT

About 1800 calories

BREAKFAST
2 pancakes

1 egg

2 pieces toast

Sugar-free pancake syrup

Coffee

BREAKFAST
$1^1/_2$ cup dry cereal

1 cup 1% milk

2 tablespoons raisins

Tea

LUNCH
Sandwich (2 slices bread, 2 ounces roast beef)

Green salad with 2 tablespoons fat-free or light salad dressing

1 apple

2 low-fat cookies

Diet soda pop

LUNCH
Fast food hamburger ($^1/_4$ pound with lettuce and tomato, no sauce)

Small fries

Diet soda pop

DINNER
Chicken stir-fry (3 ounces of chicken, vegetables)

1 cup rice

1 piece fresh fruit

Tea

DINNER
4 ounces steak

1 medium baked potato

1 dinner roll

Tossed salad with 1 tablespoon fat-free or light salad dressing

1 cup mixed vegetables

1 tablespoon margarine and 1 tablespoon light sour cream

1 cup low-fat milk

SNACK IDEAS (CHOOSE ONE)
2 pieces toast, 1 tablespoon peanut butter

1 cup cereal, 1 cup skim milk

1 cup mixed fresh fruit

Learning Resources

BOOKS
The following publications are available from IDC Publishing. For a free catalog, call (888) 637-2675.

Managing Type 2 Diabetes by Arlene Monk RD, CDE; Jan Pearson, BAN, RN, CDE; Priscilla Hollander, MD, PhD; Richard Bergenstal, MD
Managing Type 2 Diabetes is the perfect follow-up to Type 2 Diabetes BASICS. It is a comprehensive guide to self-care and health care for type 2 diabetes. It includes all the information and tools you need to take charge of your health. Complete with simple tables and charts to guide daily decisions, this easy-to-use book addresses your concerns, answers your questions, and helps you live well with diabetes.

Fast Food Facts by Marion J. Franz, MS, RD, CDE
As a definitive guide to survival in the fast-food jungle, *Fast Food Facts* shows you how to make wise selections at the top 40 fast food chains. Includes meal exchanges, "smart meals" and carbohydrate choices. Also available in a pocket edition.

Exchanges for All Occasions by Marion J. Franz, MS, RD, CDE
Completely updated and reorganized, *Exchanges for All Occasions* offers sample menus and comprehensive food lists that demonstrate how you can include a variety of foods in a healthy diet. With this book as your guide, you can enjoy all your favorite foods and stay healthy. Also available in a pocket edition.

The Convenience Foods Cookbook by Nancy Cooper, RD, CDE
Turn brand-name foods into brand-new meals! Recipes in
The Convenience Foods Cookbook transform packaged
goods into healthy dishes. Go from package to plate in just
under 20 minutes!

Convenience Food Facts by Arlene Monk RD, CDE;
Nancy Cooper, RD, CDE
Arranged for ease of comparison-shopping, *Convenience
Food Facts* guides readers to low-fat choices among more
than 3,000 popular brand-name products. In addition, the
book lists exchange values and carbohydrate choices—information not found on food labels.

DIABETES ASSOCIATIONS/CENTERS

International Diabetes Center Affiliate Network
3800 Park Nicollet Boulevard, Minneapolis, MN 55416-2699,
(888) 825-6315, www.idcdiabetes.org

American Diabetes Association 1701 North Beauregard
Street, Alexandria, VA 22311, (800) 232-3472,
www.diabetes.org

Canadian Diabetes Association 15 Toronto Street,
Suite 800, Toronto, ON M5C 2E3, Canada, (416) 363-3373,
www.diabetes.ca

DIABETES HEALTHCARE SOURCES

American Association of Diabetes Educators 100 West Monroe, Suite 400, Chicago, IL 60603, (800) 338-3633, www.addenet.org

The American Dietetic Association 216 West Jackson, Boulevard, Suite 800, Chicago, IL 60606, (800) 366-1655, www.eatright.org

American Board of Podiatric Surgery 3330 Mission Street, San Francisco, CA 94110-5009, (415) 826-3200, www.abps.org

Impotence World Association PO Box 410, Bowie, MD 20718-0410, (800) 669-1603, www.impotenceworld.org

National Eye Care Project PO Box 429098, San Francisco, CA 94142-9098, (800) 222-3937, www.eyenet.org

DIABETES MAGAZINES

Diabetes Forecast, American Diabetes Association , 1701 North Beauregard Street, Alexandria, VA 22311, www.diabetes.org/diabetesforecast

Diabetes in the News, Ames Company, Division, Miles Laboratory, Inc., PO Box 3105, Elkhart, IN 46515

Diabetes Self-Management, PO Box 851, Farmingdale, NY 11737, (800) 234-0923, www.diabetes-self-mgmt.com

ADDITIONAL DIABETES SITES ON THE INTERNET

www.onhealth.com This site has a "medical center" devoted to diabetes that is presented by the International Diabetes Center.

www.diabetesnet.com Offers general information about diabetes.

www.niddk.nih.gov/ National Institutes of Diabetes and Digestive and Kidney Diseases (National Institutes of Health)

MEDICAL IDENTIFICATION TAGS

Medical identification bracelets/necklaces are available at many department and drug stores or from these companies.

Medic Alert 2323 Colorado Avenue, Turlock, CA 95382, (800) 432-5378

Monroe Specialty Company PO Box 740, Monroe, WI 53566, (608) 328-8381

BLOOD GLUCOSE ANALYSIS SOFTWARE

In Touch LifeScan, Inc., 1000 Gibraltar, Milpitas, CA 95035, (800) 227-8862, www.lifescan.com

Mellitus Manager Metamedix, Inc., 735 East Ohio Ave, Suite 202, Escondido, CA 92025, or download a free copy of Mellitus Manager at www.metamedix.com

Camit Roche Diagnostics, (800) 858-8072, www.roche.com/diagnostics/

PrecisionLink Abbott/Medisense, Abbott Laboratories, Medisense Product Line, 4A Crosby Drive, Bedford, MA 01730-1402, (800) 527-3339 www.abbott.com

Win Glucofacts Bayer Corporation-Diagnostics, (800) 348-8100, www.bayerdiag.com

Glossary

Blood Glucose Level The amount of glucose in the blood measured by a laboratory or self blood test.

Carbohydrate Nutrient in food that comes primarily from starch and sugar. Carbohydrate is broken down into glucose for energy.

Carbohydrate Choice A measure used in carbohydrate counting. One carbohydrate choice is equal to 15 grams of carbohydrate.

Carbohydrate Counting A food planning method based on eating a set amount of carbohydrate at each meal and snack.

Cholesterol A fat-like substance that is both found in food and made by the body. High blood cholesterol is a risk for heart disease.

Food Plan An individualized schedule of meals and snacks created to help a person with diabetes maintain a target blood glucose level and proper nutrition.

Glucose A sugar made in the body when food is digested. It is the body's main source of energy.

HDL (high-density lipoprotein) A small "packet" that carries cholesterol out of arteries. A high level of HDL, often referred to as "good" cholesterol, protects against heart disease.

Hemoglobin A$_{1c}$ (HbA$_{1c}$) A blood test that shows the average blood glucose level over the last two months. It is used to evaluate diabetes control and to determine whether changes need to be made in a person's diabetes treatment plan.

Hyperglycemia A condition that occurs when the blood glucose level is higher than normal.

Hypoglycemia A condition that occurs when the blood glucose level drops too low.

Impaired Fasting Glucose or Impaired Glucose Tolerance Conditions in which a person's plasma blood glucose level is higher than normal but not high enough to be diagnosed as diabetes. Both conditions signal that the person is at risk for developing diabetes.

Insulin A hormone produced in the pancreas that allows glucose to get into cells. Without it glucose cannot be used for energy.

Ketones A potentially harmful waste product created when the body breaks down fat for energy.

LDL (low-density lipoprotein) A small "packet" that carries cholesterol and deposits it in blood vessels, which can clog them. A high level of LDL cholesterol increases the risk of heart disease, so LDL is often referred to as "bad" cholesterol.

Meter A small machine used to measure the level of glucose in blood.

Pancreas A gland located near the stomach that makes insulin.

Test Strips Chemically-treated paper or plastic strips used for self blood glucose testing.

Triglycerides Fats that are both found in food and made by the body. High triglyceride levels increase the risk for heart disease.

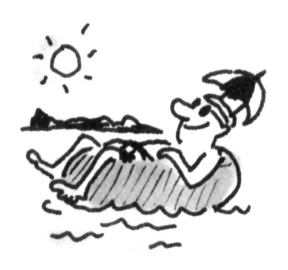